Canine Vagus Nerve Activation

Simple Ways to Boost Your Dog's Health and Happiness

Second Edition

Copyright

© 2025

All rights reserved. No part of this book may be reproduced, stored in a retrieval system, or transmitted in any form or by any means, electronic, mechanical, photocopying, recording, or otherwise, without the prior written permission of the author or publisher, except for brief quotations used in reviews or scholarly works.

For permissions or inquiries, contact:
InkedEmotionsNikky@gmail.com

Website

https://payhip.com/INKEDEMOTIONS

About This Edition

Why Choose the Second Edition?

If you're new to Canine Vagus Nerve Activation, this second edition is the most complete, up-to-date resource available. It includes everything from the first edition—like essential techniques in touch, breathing, and nutrition—but also much more.

What's new and improved?

Brand-new chapters on sound and vibration therapy, exercise for vagus nerve health, and technology-based stimulation.

In-depth guidance on heart rate variability (HRV), a cutting-edge tool for monitoring your dog's calm and stress levels.

Practical advice for creating a vagus-friendly environment that supports your dog's natural healing every day.

Expanded troubleshooting tips and real-world case studies to help you navigate challenges with confidence.

A helpful bonus section packed with actionable tips you won't find in the first edition.

If you already own the first edition, the second offers a meaningful upgrade that reflects the latest science and a broader, more holistic approach to your dog's well-being. If you're deciding which edition to buy, this version will give you the freshest insights and the most tools to support your dog's health and happiness.

In short:
First edition = great foundation.
Second edition = deeper, wider, and smarter support for you and your dog.

Welcome to a new journey of calm, connection, and healing.

Nikky

Table of Contents

Copyright

About This Edition:
Why Choose the Second Edition?

Table of Contents

Disclaimer

Dedication

Why I Wrote This Book

About the Author

Before We Begin

Note on Scientific References

Chapter One
What Is the Vagus Nerve and Why It Matters to Your Dog

Chapter Two
Recognizing Vagal Tone in Dogs

Chapter Three
The Gut-Brain Axis in Dogs

Chapter Four
Daily Habits to Improve Vagal Tone

Chapter Five
The Power of Breath and Touch

Chapter Six
Canine Massage Techniques for Vagal Activation

Chapter Seven

Using Sound and Vibration

Chapter Eight
Nutrition and the Vagal Connection

Chapter Nine
The Role of Exercise in Vagus Nerve Health

Chapter Ten
Managing Stress and Anxiety with Vagal Activation

Chapter Eleven
Technology and Vagus Nerve Stimulation

Chapter Twelve
Building a Vagus-Friendly Environment

Chapter Thirteen
Case Studies and Success Stories

Chapter Fourteen
Troubleshooting and When to Seek Help

Chapter Fifteen
Heart Rate Variability (HRV) and Canine Calm

Chapter Sixteen
Breathing and Heart Rate

Conclusion
Embracing Your Dog's Natural Healing Power

Bonus Section
Practical Tips to Support Your Dog's Vagus Nerve and Well-Being

Thank You

Disclaimer

The information provided in this book is for educational and informational purposes only. It is not intended to replace professional veterinary advice, diagnosis, or treatment. Always consult your veterinarian before making any changes to your dog's health care routine, diet, or exercise program.

While the techniques and suggestions shared here have helped many dogs, individual results may vary. The author and publisher assume no responsibility or liability for any injury, illness, or adverse effects resulting from the use or misuse of the information contained in this book.

Your dog's health and well-being are important—please use this book as a helpful guide, not a substitute for professional care.

Dedication

This book is lovingly dedicated to all the dog owners, trainers, caregivers, and animal advocates who tirelessly seek to deepen the connection with their canine companions. Your patience, kindness, and dedication to understanding your dogs go beyond words. You see them not just as pets, but as family members, teachers, and soul friends.

To every dog who has ever waited patiently for a kind touch, a comforting word, or a moment of calm in a busy world—you are the true heroes of this journey. Your resilience, your unwavering loyalty, and your capacity to teach us about unconditional love inspire everything within these pages.

I also dedicate this book to those dogs who have faced challenges—whether physical, emotional, or behavioral—and to the humans who never gave up on them. Together, you embody hope, healing, and transformation.

May this work serve as a bridge, helping to deepen the trust, joy, and well-being between humans and their dogs. May it remind us all to listen more closely, touch more gently, breathe more mindfully, and nurture more compassionately.

Thank you for being part of this journey of healing and connection.

Why I Wrote This Book

For over 23 years, I have poured my heart and soul into running a non-profit dog rescue, Save a Dog Today. Through this journey, I've cared for three different packs of dogs—18 in total—each with their own stories, struggles, and incredible spirits. These dogs weren't just rescues; they became my family, my teachers, and my motivation to understand canine health on a deeper level.

Living with and caring for dogs who were often overlooked or unwanted showed me how deeply stress, trauma, and emotional wounds affect their behavior and well-being. I saw how much more they needed than food and shelter—they needed connection, calm, and healing from the inside out.

This sparked my passion for exploring natural, science-based ways to help dogs thrive. That's how I came to focus on the vagus nerve, an amazing part of the nervous system that influences everything from a dog's digestion to their emotional balance. Unlocking the power of vagal activation felt like discovering a missing link—a way to support dogs not just physically, but emotionally and mentally too.

I wrote this book to share what I've learned with other dog lovers who want to give their companions the very best in health and happiness. It's a guide born from decades of hands-on experience, deep care, and a desire to see every dog live a peaceful, joyful life.

If you've ever loved a dog like family, if you've ever wished for a deeper connection and a way to ease their stress and anxiety, this book is for you. Together, we can unlock the natural healing power that lives within every dog's body and heart.

About the Author

Nikky Rich is a devoted animal lover, writer, and health advocate with over two decades of experience dedicated to health and wellness—not only for herself but for humans, family, and animals alike. For more than 23 years, she has run the non-profit dog rescue Save a Dog Today, where she personally cared for 18 dogs in her own home—dogs who either couldn't find the right adoptive family or were considered not adoptable. These 18 dogs became lifelong members of her family, forming three loving packs under her care.

This number does not include the many foster dogs she has opened her home to over the years, nor the hundreds of dogs she has trained, worked with, and helped throughout her rescue experience. In total, Nikky has touched the lives of hundreds, if not thousands, of dogs, bringing them safety, healing, and hope.

Nikky's deep connection to these dogs and her extensive experience sparked her passion to explore natural, science-based ways to support their health and well-being.

Before You Begin

Welcome, and thank you for choosing this book to learn about the powerful role of the vagus nerve in your dog's health and happiness. If you're eager to take your knowledge even further and gain hands-on guidance, I invite you to check out my Canine Vagus Nerve Activation Course on my website. This course is designed to walk you through practical techniques with clear demonstrations, helping you confidently support your dog's nervous system every day.

As a special thank you for purchasing this book, you qualify for a 10% discount on the course.

Website:
https://payhip.com/INKEDEMOTIONS

Simply use the promo code 13OKG2SNDZ at checkout to access this offer.
I'm excited to support you and your furry friend on this journey toward greater calm, resilience, and joy.

Now, let's get started!

Note on Scientific References

At the time of writing, all scientific links and references included in this book were active and fully functional. However, websites and databases occasionally update or remove content. If you encounter a broken link, we encourage you to search for the study title or PMID (PubMed ID) in a trusted scientific database such as PubMed to access the most current version.

Chapter One

What Is the Vagus Nerve and Why It Matters to Your Dog

When we think about our dog's health, it's natural to focus on their food, exercise, vaccinations, and regular vet visits. But beneath the surface of these visible aspects lies a vital nerve that quietly influences almost every part of your dog's physical and emotional well-being: the vagus nerve.

The vagus nerve is the tenth cranial nerve—the longest and most complex nerve in the body. It originates in the brainstem and extends through the neck into the chest and abdomen, branching out to connect with critical organs such as the heart, lungs, liver, and most importantly, the digestive tract. This nerve acts like a superhighway of communication, sending signals back and forth between the brain and the body, regulating essential functions such as heart rate, breathing, digestion, immune response, and even mood.

Why is this nerve so important? Because it is the main component of the parasympathetic nervous system, often called the "rest and digest" system. When activated, the vagus nerve promotes a state of calm by slowing the heart rate, stimulating digestive enzymes, reducing inflammation, and encouraging relaxation. This balance is crucial for your dog's ability to handle stress, recover from illness, and maintain overall health.

In scientific terms, the strength and responsiveness of the vagus nerve are measured as "vagal tone." A high vagal tone indicates a healthy, flexible nervous system capable of adapting to stress and maintaining internal balance. Conversely, a low vagal tone is linked to increased anxiety, digestive problems, poor immune function, and behavioral issues.

Scientific Insight: In mammals, including dogs, vagal tone influences many physiological and emotional processes. Breuer and Weitz (2021) explain that vagal pathways regulate autonomic control over the heart and digestive tract, playing a key role in homeostasis and emotional regulation. You can read their research here:
https://link.springer.com/article/10.1007/s00359-021-01507-9

Another important concept is the gut-brain axis, a communication network between the digestive system and the brain, heavily influenced by the vagus nerve. This explains why digestive health and emotional well-being are often linked in dogs. An imbalanced vagus nerve can disrupt digestion and create a cascade of stress responses.

Scientific Insight: Stephen Porges' Polyvagal Theory sheds light on how the vagus nerve affects emotional regulation and social engagement behaviors. His work shows that stimulating the vagus nerve can reduce anxiety-like behaviors and improve gastrointestinal function in animals. You can explore his study here: https://www.ncbi.nlm.nih.gov/pmc/articles/PMC5524082/

In practical terms, a dog with a healthy vagus nerve can better regulate stress responses, showing calmer behavior, improved digestion, and a stronger immune system. When the vagus nerve is not functioning well—due to chronic stress, trauma, illness, or injury—dogs may show signs of anxiety, digestive upset, lowered resilience, and behavior changes such as excessive barking or withdrawal.

Understanding the vagus nerve's role is the foundation of helping your dog achieve a balanced nervous system. By learning how to activate and support this nerve naturally, through breath, touch, nutrition, and more, you can unlock your dog's innate ability to heal and thrive.

In the chapters ahead, we will explore the anatomy and function of the vagus nerve in greater depth, examine how to recognize healthy vagal tone, and introduce practical, science-backed methods to enhance your dog's nervous system health.

Chapter Two

Recognizing Vagal Tone in Dogs

Understanding and recognizing your dog's vagal tone is the key to knowing how well their nervous system supports their health, behavior, and emotional resilience. Vagal tone refers to the activity and responsiveness of the vagus nerve—the higher the tone, the better the nerve can regulate critical bodily functions and calm stress responses.

What Is Vagal Tone?

Vagal tone measures the influence of the vagus nerve on the heart, lungs, and digestive system. It reflects how flexibly the nervous system can shift between states of calm ("rest and digest") and alertness ("fight or flight"). A high vagal tone means your dog's parasympathetic nervous system is strong, promoting relaxation, efficient digestion, and balanced emotional states. Low vagal tone often correlates with chronic stress, anxiety, digestive issues, and difficulty calming down after excitement or fear.

Signs of Healthy Vagal Tone in Dogs

Calm and relaxed demeanor during everyday life

Normal, steady breathing patterns (not shallow or rapid)

Good digestion and regular bowel movements without signs of discomfort

Ability to recover quickly from stress or excitement

Balanced heart rate with normal variability

Sociable and engaged behavior without excessive fear or aggression

Signs of Low Vagal Tone in Dogs

Excessive barking, whining, or restlessness

Digestive problems such as diarrhea, constipation, or bloating

Panting or rapid breathing when not hot or exercising

Difficulty settling after excitement or stressful events

Excessive anxiety or fearfulness

Poor immune response, frequent illness, or slow recovery

Measuring Vagal Tone: Heart Rate Variability (HRV)

One of the most reliable ways to assess vagal tone is by measuring heart rate variability (HRV)—the natural variation in the time interval between heartbeats. Higher HRV is a marker of greater parasympathetic (vagal) activity and better nervous system flexibility. Although this is commonly used in humans, research shows HRV can also be measured in dogs as an indicator of stress and health.

Scientific Insight: A study by Von Borell et al. (2007) highlights that HRV analysis in dogs provides valuable insight into their stress levels and emotional states. You can read the paper here:
https://www.ncbi.nlm.nih.gov/pmc/articles/PMC2249561/

Practical Observations for Dog Owners

While devices to measure HRV in dogs are emerging, most dog owners rely on behavior and physical cues. Notice how your dog responds to new environments, loud noises, or interactions with other animals. A dog with a good vagal tone will recover faster from stress and remain calm in situations that would overwhelm others.

Improving Vagal Tone

The good news is that vagal tone is not fixed. It can be improved through practices like gentle touch, controlled breathing, calming routines, proper nutrition, and regular, moderate exercise—all topics we will explore in later chapters.

Chapter Three

The Gut-Brain Axis in Dogs

When we think about a dog's health, digestion often comes to mind, but the gut's role extends far beyond breaking down food. The gut is a central player in your dog's emotional well-being and overall health, thanks to a fascinating and complex system called the gut-brain axis. This network of communication between the gut and the brain influences how your dog feels, behaves, and even how their body fights illness.

The Gut-Brain Axis: An Overview

The gut-brain axis is a sophisticated, two-way communication system linking the gastrointestinal tract and the central nervous system. At the heart of this dialogue is the vagus nerve, which carries signals in both directions—from the gut to the brain and from the brain back to the gut. These signals help regulate digestion, immune response, mood, and even cognitive functions.

In dogs, this connection is especially critical because stress, anxiety, and behavioral issues often show up alongside digestive problems. The vagus nerve acts as the messenger, translating gut conditions into neurological responses and vice versa.

The Microbiome: The Ecosystem Within

Within your dog's digestive tract lives an entire ecosystem of microorganisms—collectively known as the gut microbiota. These microscopic residents include bacteria, fungi, and viruses that play essential roles in digestion, nutrient absorption, and immune defense.

But their influence goes beyond the gut. These microbes produce neurotransmitters and metabolites that affect the brain and nervous system. For example, certain bacteria produce serotonin, often called the "feel-good" neurotransmitter, which is crucial in regulating mood and anxiety. A balanced microbiome promotes a healthy gut-brain axis and robust vagal nerve function, supporting calmness and resilience in your dog.

On the other hand, when the microbiome is disrupted—a condition called dysbiosis—it can trigger inflammation, weaken the immune system, and impair the vagus nerve's ability to regulate bodily functions. This disruption often manifests as gastrointestinal issues such as diarrhea, constipation, or bloating, alongside behavioral symptoms like irritability, restlessness, or anxiety.

The Vagus Nerve as the Communication Highway

The vagus nerve is the main conduit of the gut-brain axis. It not only sends sensory information about the gut's condition to the brain but also conveys signals that regulate digestion and inflammation. Through this bidirectional communication, the vagus nerve helps maintain homeostasis—the body's balanced internal state.

Research has revealed that vagal pathways can influence mood, stress responses, and cognitive function by modulating neurotransmitter levels and reducing systemic inflammation. In essence, the vagus nerve helps your dog's brain and body "talk" to each other to stay healthy and calm.

Scientific Evidence Supporting the Gut-Brain Axis

A growing body of scientific research underscores the importance of the gut-brain axis and the vagus nerve's role within it. For instance, a comprehensive review by Cryan and Dinan (2017) highlights how gut microbes affect brain chemistry and behavior through vagal pathways and immune signaling. Their work suggests that changes in the gut microbiota can influence anxiety, depression, and cognitive function.

You can access the study here:
https://pubmed.ncbi.nlm.nih.gov/28482030/

This research is foundational in understanding why gut health is not just about digestion—it's a cornerstone of emotional and neurological health in dogs as well as humans.

Implications for Canine Health and Behavior

When the gut-brain axis is functioning optimally, your dog benefits from improved digestion, better stress management, and a more stable mood. However, disruptions in this system can create a cascade of problems. Chronic stress or illness can alter the gut microbiota, which in turn impacts vagal nerve signaling, potentially leading to a vicious cycle of poor digestion and increased anxiety.

Recognizing the signs of gut imbalance alongside behavioral changes is essential. For example, a dog suffering from frequent diarrhea or constipation might also show signs of nervousness or irritability. These symptoms are often connected, pointing to the underlying gut-brain axis disruption.

Understanding this link opens the door to new ways of supporting your dog's health—beyond traditional treatments—by targeting the gut microbiome and nervous system to restore balance and promote overall wellness.

Chapter Four

Daily Habits to Improve Vagal Tone

Vagal tone, which reflects the activity of the vagus nerve, is not fixed — it can be nurtured and improved through simple, consistent daily habits. Building routines that promote calmness and reduce stress can strengthen your dog's parasympathetic nervous system, improving emotional resilience, digestion, immune function, and overall well-being.

This chapter explores practical daily habits that support your dog's vagal tone and foster a balanced nervous system.

The Power of Routine

Dogs are creatures of habit. Predictable daily schedules help regulate their internal clock and nervous system by providing a sense of safety and control. When dogs know what to expect, their stress hormone levels (like cortisol) decrease, and vagal tone improves.

For example, feeding your dog at the same time every day supports digestive regularity and gut health — both closely linked to the vagus nerve. Consistent feeding routines also reduce anxiety around food and meal anticipation.

Structured Exercise and Walks

Physical activity isn't just for fitness; it's a vital tool for vagal activation. Regular, moderate exercise boosts parasympathetic activity post-workout, increasing heart rate variability and promoting relaxation.

Walks serve multiple purposes: they provide mental stimulation, social interaction, and a controlled outlet for energy. Predictable walk times and routes give your dog a comforting structure, reducing hypervigilance and stress.

Vagal tone benefits most when walks are calm and rhythmic, avoiding overstimulation from chaotic environments or uncontrolled excitement.

Loving Touch and Social Connection

Daily affectionate touch, such as gentle petting, brushing, or massage, engages sensory receptors that activate the vagus nerve. This tactile stimulation reduces heart rate and cortisol, increasing relaxation and strengthening the bond between you and your dog.

Social interaction with trusted humans and other dogs also influences vagal tone. Positive play and calm companionship boost oxytocin release and vagal activity, which supports emotional stability.

Mindful Rest and Quiet Time

Providing your dog with a calm, quiet space for rest is essential. Just like humans, dogs need downtime to reset their nervous system. Quality sleep and relaxation periods support the vagus nerve by allowing the body's parasympathetic system to dominate.

Minimizing sudden loud noises, chaotic activity, and excessive stimulation during rest times helps maintain this calm.

Consistency Builds Calm

Incorporating these habits into a daily routine isn't about perfection—it's about consistency and predictability. Over time, these small rituals accumulate, increasing vagal tone and your dog's ability to self-regulate stress.

Dogs thrive when they feel safe, connected, and understood. Your daily actions are the foundation of that safety.

Scientific Snippet:
Daily routines reduce stress hormone levels and stabilize the autonomic nervous system, supporting vagal tone and emotional balance.
https://www.ncbi.nlm.nih.gov/pmc/articles/PMC6335198/

These daily habits are simple to start and profoundly impactful. They support your dog's natural ability to relax and thrive by nurturing the vagus nerve, the body's built-in healing and calming system.

Chapter Five

The Power of Breath and Touch

Breathing is a subtle yet powerful way to influence the vagus nerve and the autonomic nervous system—not only in humans but in dogs as well. While dogs breathe naturally, the rhythm and quality of their breath closely reflect their emotional state. By intentionally using your own calm, steady breath alongside gentle, loving touch, you can help your dog shift from a state of stress or arousal into deep relaxation and parasympathetic dominance.

Breath as a Bridge to Calm

The vagus nerve acts as a bridge between the brain and body, regulating heart rate, digestion, and emotional balance. Slow, diaphragmatic (belly) breathing activates the vagus nerve by stimulating sensory receptors in the lungs and diaphragm. This leads to a cascade of calming physiological effects, including lowered heart rate and increased heart rate variability (HRV).

Though dogs cannot consciously control their breath like humans, they instinctively mirror the emotional cues of their owners. When you breathe slowly and calmly near your dog, their nervous system can follow your lead, helping to entrain their breath toward a more relaxed pattern.

The Role of Touch in Vagal Activation

Touch works synergistically with breath to influence the vagus nerve. Gentle petting, stroking, or massage stimulates sensory receptors in the skin and muscles that send calming signals to the brainstem, where the vagus nerve originates.

This tactile stimulation reduces stress hormones such as cortisol, promotes oxytocin release (the bonding hormone), and lowers sympathetic nervous system activity. Touch offers an immediate physical connection that supports your dog's emotional security and helps regulate their nervous system.

Creating Breath and Touch Moments

Mirroring Breath: Sit or lie calmly with your dog and consciously slow your breath. Breathe deeply into your belly with a smooth, even rhythm. As you do, gently stroke your dog's chest, neck, or back in sync with your exhale. This combination creates a powerful calming signal.

Rhythmic Touch: Use slow, repetitive strokes or gentle massage to reinforce parasympathetic activation. Focus on areas rich in vagus nerve branches such as the neck, chest, abdomen, and base of the ears.

Consistent Practice: These moments don't have to be long. Even five minutes of intentional breathing paired with touch can shift your dog's nervous system toward calm. With consistent practice, your dog's baseline vagal tone improves.

Scientific Evidence

Studies show that slow diaphragmatic breathing stimulates the vagus nerve, reducing heart rate and increasing HRV, which correlates with improved emotional regulation and stress resilience. This effect has been documented in humans and mammals generally, providing a solid foundation for applying breath-based calming to dogs.

Scientific Snippet:
Slow diaphragmatic breathing stimulates the vagus nerve, reducing heart rate and increasing heart rate variability.
https://www.ncbi.nlm.nih.gov/pmc/articles/PMC5709795/

Why Breath and Touch Matter

Together, breath and touch offer a non-invasive, accessible way to activate the vagus nerve and support your dog's health on multiple levels. This natural combination promotes relaxation, improves digestion, balances the immune system, and strengthens the emotional bond between you and your dog.

By regularly incorporating breath and touch into your daily routine, you are nurturing your dog's nervous system resilience and helping them navigate life's stresses with greater ease and calm.

Chapter Six

Canine Massage Techniques for Vagal Activation

Massage is a powerful, hands-on way to stimulate the vagus nerve in your dog, helping to calm anxiety, reduce heart rate, and improve overall parasympathetic function. By engaging specific areas rich in vagal nerve fibers, you can encourage your dog's nervous system to shift from fight-or-flight to rest-and-digest mode. This chapter provides detailed, safe, and effective massage techniques designed to activate the vagus nerve and promote deep relaxation.

Why Massage Stimulates the Vagus Nerve

The vagus nerve has branches that run through the ears, neck, chest, and abdomen. Gentle stimulation of these areas sends calming sensory input to the brainstem, triggering the parasympathetic nervous system. This leads to a reduction in cortisol (stress hormone), increased release of oxytocin (the bonding hormone), slower heart rate, and improved digestion.

Massage also helps release muscle tension and increases blood flow, which together support your dog's physical comfort and emotional well-being.

Step-by-Step Massage Protocols for Vagal Activation

1. Ear Stroking
The external ear (auricle) contains branches of the vagus nerve, making it an ideal place to begin. Use your fingertips to gently stroke the base and edges of your dog's ears in slow, circular motions. Start with light pressure, increasing slightly if your dog enjoys it. This technique is soothing and can quickly reduce anxiety.

2. Neck and Shoulder Massage
Place your hands on either side of your dog's neck and use long, gentle strokes downward toward the shoulders. This area houses many vagus nerve fibers and muscle tension spots. Massage slowly and rhythmically, paying attention to your dog's reactions to ensure comfort.

3. Chest and Sternum Massage
Using your palms or fingertips, apply gentle circular motions over the chest and sternum area. This stimulates the vagus nerve pathways and helps regulate heart rate and breathing. Some dogs may be sensitive here, so proceed carefully and stop if your dog shows discomfort.

4. Abdominal Massage
Light, clockwise circular strokes on the abdomen support digestion and vagal tone through the gut-brain axis. Use soft pressure and observe your dog's cues. Abdominal massage can relieve tension and improve gastrointestinal motility.

When and How Often to Massage

Massage sessions can be brief—5 to 10 minutes daily or a few times a week—depending on your dog's tolerance and needs. The best times are during calm moments, after exercise, or in anticipation of potentially stressful events like vet visits or thunderstorms.

Consistency helps build and maintain a strong vagal tone over time. Be patient and responsive to your dog's comfort, making massage a positive and bonding experience.

Safety and Comfort Tips

Always start with gentle pressure and adjust based on your dog's feedback.

Avoid areas with injury, inflammation, or extreme sensitivity without veterinary guidance.

Use a calm voice and soothing presence to enhance the relaxation effect.

Combine massage with slow breathing to deepen vagal activation.

Scientific Evidence

Auricular vagus nerve stimulation (aVNS)—stimulation of the ear's vagal branches—has been shown to improve parasympathetic function, reducing heart rate and anxiety in mammals. This non-invasive technique is safe and effective for enhancing vagal tone and emotional regulation.

Scientific Snippet:
Auricular vagus nerve stimulation (aVNS) improves parasympathetic function and reduces anxiety.
https://pubmed.ncbi.nlm.nih.gov/33159864/

Massage is a simple yet profound way to tap into your dog's natural healing system. With mindful touch and consistency, you can help your dog access the calming power of the vagus nerve, leading to better health, mood, and connection.

Chapter Seven

Using Sound and Vibration

Sound and vibration have long been recognized as powerful tools for influencing the nervous system, and modern science is uncovering their specific effects on the vagus nerve. Certain sounds—ranging from soothing music to targeted acoustic frequencies—can resonate with the body's natural rhythms, stimulating vagal pathways and promoting relaxation, emotional balance, and healing in dogs.

This chapter explores how sound and vibration can be used intentionally to support your dog's nervous system health and vagal tone.

How Sound Affects the Vagus Nerve

The vagus nerve contains sensory fibers connected to the ear and throat, making it responsive to acoustic stimuli. When exposed to calming, rhythmic sounds or specific frequencies, these fibers send signals to the brainstem that enhance parasympathetic activity, lowering heart rate, reducing cortisol levels, and increasing heart rate variability (HRV).

Acoustic stimulation influences brainwave patterns and mood-related biomarkers, helping dogs—and humans—enter states of calm and focused relaxation. This is why sound therapy has gained popularity as a non-invasive method to manage anxiety, stress, and even pain.

Therapeutic Sounds and Frequencies

Singing Bowls and Tuning Forks: These instruments produce sustained harmonic vibrations that resonate with the body's natural frequencies. The gentle, steady tones encourage relaxation and vagal activation.

Low-Frequency Sounds (20–500 Hz): Research suggests that low-frequency acoustic waves are particularly effective at stimulating the vagus nerve. These frequencies mimic the natural rhythms of the heart and breath, helping to synchronize nervous system activity.

White Noise and Nature Sounds: Gentle background sounds like rain, ocean waves, or forest ambiance can mask disruptive noises, creating a safe, soothing soundscape that supports parasympathetic dominance.

Music with Slow Tempo: Music at around 60–80 beats per minute aligns closely with resting heart rates, promoting calm and aiding vagal tone enhancement.

Creating a Healing Soundscape for Your Dog

Select instruments or recordings that produce gentle, rhythmic sounds with no sudden changes in volume or pitch.

Play sounds at a comfortable volume, ensuring they do not startle or overwhelm your dog.

Use sound therapy sessions during rest periods, vet visits, or stressful situations like fireworks or travel.

Combine sound with other calming techniques such as massage or slow breathing for a holistic approach.

Scientific Evidence

Acoustic stimulation has been shown to activate vagal pathways and improve mood-related biomarkers in mammals. The effects include decreased anxiety, improved emotional regulation, and enhanced autonomic balance.

Scientific Snippet:
Acoustic stimulation activates vagal pathways and improves mood-related biomarkers.
https://www.frontiersin.org/articles/10.3389/fpsyt.2020.00370/full

Why Sound and Vibration Matter

Sound and vibration offer a non-invasive, easy-to-implement method to support your dog's vagus nerve health. By incorporating calming acoustic elements into your dog's environment, you can reduce stress, improve emotional well-being, and foster a deeper connection through shared peaceful experiences.

Experimenting with sound therapy can be a gentle way to help your dog navigate the challenges of modern life with greater ease and calm.

Chapter Eight

Nutrition and the Vagal Connection

Nutrition plays a fundamental role in shaping your dog's health, mood, and nervous system function—especially the vagus nerve. What your dog eats impacts gut health, systemic inflammation, and even brain chemistry, all of which influence vagal tone and parasympathetic balance. This chapter delves into dietary strategies and nutrients that support the vagus nerve and promote emotional and physical well-being.

The Gut-Vagus-Brain Axis and Diet

The gut and brain communicate bidirectionally through the vagus nerve, forming what is known as the gut-brain axis. A healthy gut microbiome—the trillions of beneficial bacteria living in the intestines—supports this communication by producing neurotransmitters, short-chain fatty acids, and other compounds that stimulate the vagus nerve and regulate mood.

Conversely, an imbalanced microbiome or chronic gut inflammation can impair vagal signaling, contributing to anxiety, digestive disorders, and systemic inflammation.

Anti-Inflammatory Diets for Vagal Tone

Chronic inflammation negatively affects vagal nerve function. Diets that reduce inflammation support vagal tone by promoting a balanced immune response and healthier gut lining.

Key components include:

Omega-3 Fatty Acids: Found in fish oil, flaxseed, and chia seeds, omega-3s reduce inflammatory markers and enhance vagus nerve signaling. They also support brain health and cognitive function.

Antioxidant-Rich Foods: Ingredients like blueberries, spinach, and turmeric contain antioxidants that combat oxidative stress, preserving nerve function.

Whole Food Ingredients: Minimally processed diets rich in vegetables, lean proteins, and healthy fats provide nutrients essential for nerve repair and function.

Probiotics and Prebiotics: Feeding the Vagus Nerve

Probiotics are beneficial bacteria that help maintain gut balance. Prebiotics are fibers that feed these good bacteria. Both play crucial roles in stimulating the vagus nerve through the gut-brain axis.

Including probiotics such as Lactobacillus and Bifidobacterium strains in your dog's diet can enhance vagal activity and reduce anxiety-like behaviors. Prebiotic fibers found in foods like chicory root, asparagus, and pumpkin help nourish these bacteria, supporting long-term gut health.

Supplements Supporting Vagal Function

Certain supplements have been shown to benefit vagus nerve function and parasympathetic balance:

Magnesium: Helps regulate nerve excitability and supports relaxation.

Vitamin B Complex: Essential for nerve health and neurotransmitter synthesis.

Herbal Adaptogens: Such as ashwagandha and holy basil may reduce stress and support nervous system balance (consult a vet before use).

Always introduce supplements under veterinary guidance, considering your dog's individual health needs.

Scientific Evidence

Diets rich in omega-3 fatty acids and probiotics have been shown to support vagal tone and reduce systemic inflammation, leading to improved mood and resilience in mammals.

Scientific Snippet:
Diets rich in omega-3 fatty acids and probiotics support vagal tone and reduce systemic inflammation.
https://pubmed.ncbi.nlm.nih.gov/30278834/

Why Nutrition Matters for Vagal Health

Optimal nutrition not only fuels your dog's body but also nurtures the complex neural pathways that regulate stress and emotional balance. By providing anti-inflammatory, gut-supportive foods and targeted supplements, you help maintain a healthy gut-brain axis and promote a calm, resilient nervous system.

Feeding your dog with this connection in mind can transform not just their physical health but their behavior, mood, and quality of life.

Chapter Nine

The Role of Exercise in Vagus Nerve Health

Exercise is more than just physical activity for your dog—it's a vital contributor to nervous system health, particularly in strengthening the vagus nerve and enhancing parasympathetic function. Regular, moderate exercise helps lower stress hormones like cortisol and adrenaline, while improving heart rate variability (HRV), an important marker of vagal tone and emotional resilience.

This chapter explores how exercise influences the vagus nerve and offers guidance on the best types of activities to support your dog's nervous system and overall well-being.

How Exercise Boosts Vagal Tone

When your dog exercises, the body releases endorphins and other feel-good chemicals that reduce stress and promote relaxation. Moderate exercise stimulates the parasympathetic nervous system by increasing HRV, meaning the vagus nerve is more active and responsive.

Exercise also improves cardiovascular fitness and circulation, which helps nourish nerve tissues and supports efficient vagal signaling. Regular physical activity encourages better sleep, digestion, and immune function—all processes regulated by the vagus nerve.

Types of Exercise That Support Vagus Nerve Health

Walking: Calm, rhythmic walks are ideal for activating the parasympathetic system. Walking in natural environments further reduces stress through sensory engagement with sights, sounds, and smells.

Swimming: Low-impact and soothing, swimming provides gentle resistance that promotes cardiovascular health and relaxation without joint strain.

Play: Interactive play with toys or other dogs can boost mood and social bonding, which indirectly supports vagal tone through oxytocin release.

Mindful Movement: Activities like controlled obedience training or scent work that combine physical movement with mental focus help regulate the nervous system by balancing arousal and calm.

Avoid Overexertion and Stress

While exercise is beneficial, intense or prolonged physical activity can trigger sympathetic nervous system dominance (fight-or-flight), temporarily lowering vagal tone. It's important to tailor exercise sessions to your dog's age, breed, fitness level, and temperament.

Signs that exercise might be too stressful include excessive panting, pacing, or refusal to continue. Always prioritize moderate, enjoyable activities that leave your dog feeling refreshed rather than exhausted.

Scientific Evidence

Studies show that moderate exercise increases parasympathetic activity and improves heart rate variability in animals, indicating enhanced vagal tone and stress resilience.

Scientific Snippet:
Moderate exercise increases parasympathetic activity and improves HRV in animals.
https://pubmed.ncbi.nlm.nih.gov/29201516/

Why Exercise Matters for Vagal Health

Incorporating regular, moderate exercise into your dog's routine not only improves physical fitness but also supports the nervous system's ability to self-regulate stress and maintain emotional balance. This makes your dog more resilient to challenges and contributes to a longer, healthier life.

Exercise is a natural, effective way to engage and strengthen the vagus nerve, creating a foundation for calm, well-being, and joyful living.

Chapter Ten

Managing Stress and Anxiety with Vagal Activation

Stress is one of the biggest enemies of healthy vagus nerve function. Chronic or acute stress disrupts the delicate balance of your dog's autonomic nervous system, often tipping it toward sympathetic dominance—the fight-or-flight response. This imbalance lowers vagal tone, impairs immune function, and can lead to anxiety, digestive issues, and behavioral problems.

This chapter explores practical, effective strategies to manage your dog's stress and anxiety by activating the vagus nerve and promoting parasympathetic nervous system dominance.

How Stress Impacts the Vagus Nerve

When your dog experiences stress, the body releases cortisol and adrenaline. While useful in short bursts, persistent high levels of these stress hormones damage vagal tone and reduce the body's ability to regulate inflammation and heal. This impaired vagal function can lead to heightened anxiety, poor digestion, and weakened immune defense.

Recognizing stress and intervening early with calming strategies can prevent chronic vagal dysfunction and support your dog's long-term health.

Creating a Calm Environment

Safe spaces play a crucial role in vagal activation. Designate a quiet, comfortable area in your home where your dog can retreat and feel secure. This refuge should be free from loud noises, harsh lighting, and excessive foot traffic.

Adding familiar bedding, toys, and calming scents such as lavender can enhance this space's soothing effect. Encouraging your dog to use this area during stressful times, like thunderstorms or vet visits, helps regulate nervous system responses.

Mindfulness and Predictable Routines

Dogs benefit immensely from predictability. Consistent daily schedules for feeding, exercise, and rest reduce uncertainty and lower stress hormone levels, indirectly supporting vagal tone.

Mindfulness in your interactions means tuning into your dog's cues, speaking softly, and maintaining calm body language. These practices send safety signals to your dog's nervous system, encouraging parasympathetic activation.

Additional Calming Techniques

Slow, rhythmic petting or massage stimulates the vagus nerve through touch, reducing heart rate and anxiety.

Breathing together with slow, deep breaths can entrain your dog's nervous system toward relaxation.

Sound therapy with gentle music or nature sounds masks disruptive noise and supports calm.

Avoiding overstimulation from chaotic environments or sudden loud noises minimizes vagal suppression.

Scientific Evidence

Research shows that chronic stress decreases vagal tone and impairs immune response, underscoring the importance of managing stress to preserve your dog's health and emotional well-being.

Scientific Snippet:
Chronic stress decreases vagal tone and impairs immune response.
https://pubmed.ncbi.nlm.nih.gov/24593043/

Why Managing Stress Is Essential

Helping your dog maintain balanced vagal tone through stress management promotes not only emotional calm but also physical resilience. By building safe spaces, establishing routines, and using calming techniques, you empower your dog to navigate life's challenges with less anxiety and better health.

Stress is inevitable, but its impact can be softened with thoughtful, vagus-nerve-supportive care.

Chapter Eleven

Technology and Vagus Nerve Stimulation

Advances in technology have introduced new tools for supporting vagus nerve function, offering promising options for veterinary care. Devices designed to stimulate the vagus nerve non-invasively can help dogs suffering from chronic inflammation, anxiety, and other health challenges by restoring autonomic balance and promoting parasympathetic activation.

This chapter reviews the latest technologies available, how they work, and their potential benefits and safety considerations for canine use.

What Is Vagus Nerve Stimulation (VNS)?

Vagus nerve stimulation involves delivering mild electrical impulses or mechanical stimuli to the vagus nerve to enhance its activity. Originally developed for humans to treat epilepsy and depression, VNS has expanded into veterinary medicine as a novel approach to managing stress-related disorders, inflammatory conditions, and chronic pain.

Non-invasive VNS devices stimulate the nerve via the skin, often targeting the ear or neck regions where vagal branches are accessible.

Types of VNS Devices for Dogs

Transcutaneous Auricular VNS (taVNS): These devices deliver electrical impulses to the ear's vagal nerve branches through adhesive electrodes. taVNS is painless, portable, and can be administered at home or in clinical settings.

Mechanical or Vibrotactile Stimulators: Some devices use gentle vibrations or pressure to stimulate the vagus nerve without electrical current, offering an alternative for sensitive dogs.

Wearable Technology: Emerging wearable collars and harnesses incorporate VNS technology, combining continuous monitoring with stimulation to optimize vagal tone throughout the day.

Benefits of VNS for Dogs

Research indicates that non-invasive vagus nerve stimulation can:

Reduce anxiety and behavioral symptoms related to stress.

Decrease systemic inflammation by regulating immune responses.

Improve heart rate variability, indicating better autonomic nervous system balance.

Support recovery from chronic conditions by enhancing nervous system plasticity.

Safety and Usage Considerations

While promising, VNS technology should be used under veterinary supervision. Device settings, duration, and frequency of stimulation must be tailored to each dog's individual needs.

Not all dogs are candidates for VNS; contraindications include certain cardiac or neurological conditions. Proper training and gradual introduction are key to ensuring comfort and efficacy.

Scientific Evidence

Studies in animals demonstrate that non-invasive vagus nerve stimulation improves autonomic balance and reduces symptoms of anxiety, validating its use as a supportive therapy.

Scientific Snippet:
Non-invasive vagus nerve stimulation devices improve autonomic balance and reduce symptoms of anxiety.
https://pubmed.ncbi.nlm.nih.gov/32040801/

Looking Ahead

As technology advances, vagus nerve stimulation devices are likely to become more accessible and customizable for canine health. Integrating VNS with behavioral and medical care offers a holistic path toward managing chronic stress and inflammation.

Understanding and embracing these emerging tools can give dog owners and veterinarians new ways to harness the vagus nerve's healing power for happier, healthier dogs.

Chapter Twelve

Building a Vagus-Friendly Environment

Your dog's environment plays a vital role in shaping their nervous system health, including the activity of the vagus nerve. A calm, nurturing space reduces stress, enhances parasympathetic function, and supports emotional well-being. This chapter explores how elements like lighting, scents, sounds, and social interaction influence vagal tone and practical steps you can take to create a vagus-friendly home for your dog.

The Impact of Environment on Vagal Tone

The autonomic nervous system, which includes the vagus nerve, constantly monitors and responds to sensory input from your dog's surroundings. Stressful or chaotic environments activate the sympathetic nervous system (fight-or-flight), suppressing vagal tone and increasing anxiety and inflammation.

Conversely, environments enriched with soothing sensory cues promote parasympathetic dominance, enhancing relaxation, digestion, and immune function.

Lighting for Calmness

Soft, natural lighting or dimmable lamps help regulate circadian rhythms and reduce overstimulation. Avoid harsh fluorescent lights or sudden bright flashes that can startle and stress your dog.

Providing areas with gentle, indirect light allows your dog to rest peacefully and supports healthy sleep patterns, which are crucial for vagal tone maintenance.

Scents and Aromatherapy

Certain scents have calming effects by stimulating olfactory pathways connected to the brain and vagus nerve. Lavender, chamomile, and cedarwood are known for their soothing properties.

Using essential oils safely (diffused in well-ventilated spaces and never applied directly to your dog's skin) can create a comforting atmosphere that lowers stress hormones and supports parasympathetic activation.

Sounds and Acoustic Environment

Quiet, consistent background sounds such as soft classical music or nature sounds can mask sudden noises and create a stable auditory environment. Avoid loud or erratic sounds that disrupt nervous system balance.

Soundscapes that promote relaxation help your dog stay calm and improve vagal tone by reducing the frequency and intensity of stress responses.

Social Interaction and Companionship

Positive social engagement with trusted humans and compatible canine companions enhances oxytocin release and vagal activity. Regular, calm interactions build emotional security and resilience.

Conversely, social isolation or unpredictable interactions can elevate stress and suppress vagal tone. Ensure your dog has access to supportive relationships tailored to their personality and needs.

Enrichment and Safe Spaces

Environmental enrichment, including toys, chew items, and varied sensory experiences, provides mental stimulation without overstimulation. Safe spaces—quiet corners or cozy beds—offer retreat opportunities where your dog can relax undisturbed.

Balancing stimulation and rest within the environment encourages optimal nervous system function.

Scientific Evidence

Research demonstrates that environmental enrichment supports parasympathetic nervous system activity and promotes behavioral health in animals.

Scientific Snippet:
Environmental enrichment supports parasympathetic nervous system activity and behavioral health.
https://pubmed.ncbi.nlm.nih.gov/28342282/

Creating Your Dog's Vagus-Friendly Home

By thoughtfully adjusting lighting, scents, sounds, and social dynamics, you create a sanctuary that nurtures your dog's vagal tone and overall well-being. This environment reduces chronic stress, supports healing, and fosters a sense of safety that allows your dog to thrive physically and emotionally.

Chapter Thirteen

Case Studies and Success Stories

Understanding how vagus nerve activation can transform a dog's life is best appreciated through real-world examples. This chapter shares detailed case studies and success stories that highlight the practical benefits of vagal stimulation techniques—showcasing improvements in behavior, anxiety reduction, and overall health enhancement.

Case Study 1: Calming a Rescue Dog with Anxiety

Max, a three-year-old rescue Labrador mix, arrived at a shelter with severe anxiety—excessive barking, pacing, and poor socialization. After integrating daily vagus nerve activation practices, including gentle massage, structured walks, and sound therapy with calming music, Max's behavior began to change.

Over six weeks, his heart rate variability improved, and he showed fewer signs of distress. Max became more sociable and responsive to training, demonstrating the positive impact of vagal tone enhancement on emotional regulation.

Case Study 2: Managing Chronic Inflammation in a Senior Dog

Bella, a ten-year-old Golden Retriever with arthritis and digestive issues, was introduced to a combined protocol of dietary changes rich in omega-3 fatty acids, daily moderate exercise, and regular ear and chest massage for vagal stimulation.

Within three months, Bella showed reduced inflammation markers, improved mobility, and a calmer demeanor. Her improved digestion and sleep quality further confirmed the role of vagal nerve support in managing chronic health conditions.

Case Study 3: Easing Separation Anxiety Through Routine and Touch

Luna, a two-year-old Border Collie, suffered from severe separation anxiety, manifesting in destructive behavior and vocalization when left alone. Her owner implemented a consistent daily routine with predictable feeding times, combined with slow breathing exercises and gentle ear stroking to activate the vagus nerve.

After eight weeks, Luna's anxiety decreased significantly. She began resting calmly during alone time, and her overall stress levels dropped, demonstrating how routine and vagal activation reduce anxiety behaviors.

Scientific Evidence Supporting These Outcomes

Vagal nerve activation improves parasympathetic function, leading to reduced anxiety and enhanced immune response. The following study supports the physiological basis for these positive outcomes:

Scientific Snippet:
Vagus nerve stimulation reduces anxiety and improves autonomic regulation in mammals.
https://pubmed.ncbi.nlm.nih.gov/28088550/

Why These Stories Matter

These examples illustrate the tangible, life-changing effects of activating the vagus nerve in dogs. Each case highlights how targeted practices—whether massage, sound therapy, exercise, or nutrition—can help dogs regain emotional balance, reduce anxiety, and support healing.

By applying these techniques consistently, you can offer your dog the same pathway to improved health and happiness.

Chapter Fourteen

Troubleshooting and When to Seek Help

While vagus nerve activation techniques can provide powerful support for your dog's emotional and physical well-being, it's important to recognize when professional veterinary care is necessary. This chapter guides you in identifying warning signs that require medical attention, how to safely integrate vagal activation practices with traditional treatments, and tips for troubleshooting common challenges.

Recognizing When to Seek Veterinary Advice

Certain symptoms and situations indicate that your dog needs professional evaluation rather than solely relying on at-home vagus nerve support:

Persistent or Severe Symptoms: If your dog exhibits ongoing anxiety, aggression, chronic pain, digestive issues, or neurological symptoms that do not improve or worsen despite your efforts, veterinary assessment is crucial.

Sudden Behavioral Changes: Abrupt shifts in behavior such as withdrawal, confusion, seizures, or severe lethargy may signal underlying medical conditions requiring urgent care.

Physical Injuries or Illness: Any signs of trauma, infection, fever, vomiting, diarrhea, or mobility loss warrant immediate veterinary attention.

Medication and Condition Management: Dogs on prescribed medications or managing chronic diseases should have vagus nerve practices integrated carefully with their treatment plans to avoid conflicts or adverse effects.

Integrating Vagus Nerve Activation with Veterinary Care

Vagus nerve stimulation techniques complement rather than replace veterinary medicine. Here's how to safely combine approaches:

Consult Your Veterinarian: Before beginning any new interventions, discuss your plans with your vet, especially if your dog has a diagnosed condition or is taking medications.

Gradual Introduction: Start vagal activation practices slowly, monitoring your dog's responses. Discontinue if you notice signs of discomfort or stress.

Collaborative Approach: Share progress and observations with your veterinarian. Adjust techniques based on professional recommendations and your dog's evolving health status.

Emergency Preparedness: Always have a plan for emergencies. Vagus nerve practices are supportive but not substitutes for urgent medical care.

Troubleshooting Common Challenges

Dog Resistance: Some dogs may initially resist touch or new routines. Use positive reinforcement, patience, and gradual exposure to help them acclimate.

Overstimulation: Excessive or vigorous massage, loud sounds, or intense exercise can increase sympathetic nervous activity rather than calm it. Observe your dog closely and adjust intensity accordingly.

Inconsistent Results: Vagus nerve tone improves with consistency over time. Occasional setbacks are normal—maintain regular practice and track progress.

Identifying Individual Needs: Each dog is unique. What works well for one may not suit another. Tailor vagal techniques to your dog's personality, health, and preferences.

When Professional Help Enhances Outcomes

In cases of severe anxiety, chronic pain, neurological disorders, or immune dysfunction, specialized interventions such as veterinary behavioral therapy, acupuncture, or prescription medications may be necessary alongside vagus nerve activation.

Seeking expert guidance ensures your dog receives comprehensive care and the best chance for recovery and quality of life.

Vagus nerve activation is a valuable tool for supporting your dog's health and emotional balance. However, knowing when to seek veterinary care and how to integrate these techniques safely ensures that your dog's well-being is prioritized holistically.

By combining compassionate at-home practices with professional medical advice, you create the strongest foundation for your dog's thriving health and happiness.

Chapter Fifteen

Heart Rate Variability (HRV) and Canine Calm

Heart Rate Variability (HRV) is a critical indicator of how well a dog's autonomic nervous system—and particularly the vagus nerve—is functioning. When a dog's HRV is high, it suggests that the parasympathetic nervous system is active and effective, which means the dog is relaxed, resilient to stress, and emotionally balanced. Conversely, a low HRV can signal chronic stress, anxiety, illness, or nervous system dysregulation.

Understanding HRV in Dogs

HRV refers to the tiny fluctuations in time between each heartbeat. These changes are not random—they reflect how well the nervous system is responding to both internal and external stimuli. The vagus nerve plays a key role here: when it's stimulated appropriately, it sends calming signals to the heart via the parasympathetic system, which improves HRV and helps a dog stay in a calm, regulated state.

A well-functioning vagus nerve allows for adaptive shifts in HRV throughout the day. For instance, during sleep or rest, the HRV should be higher, while moments of activity or arousal might see temporary decreases. The healthier and more responsive the vagus nerve, the better the overall HRV pattern—and the calmer and more behaviorally resilient the dog becomes.

HRV as a Window into Stress Resilience

HRV gives us a measurable way to understand a dog's stress resilience. Veterinarians and researchers now use wearable technology or specialized veterinary HRV monitors to track HRV in dogs during recovery from illness, stress-related conditions, or training programs designed to promote calmness.

How Can You Check Your Dog's HRV?

While HRV monitors designed specifically for dogs are not as widespread as those for humans, there are devices and methods you can explore:

Wearable Veterinary Monitors: Some veterinary clinics use specialized ECG or heart rate monitors to measure HRV in dogs. These are professional tools but increasingly accessible.

Pet-Specific Fitness Trackers: Products like the PetPace Collar monitor vital signs, including heart rate and HRV, providing real-time data on your dog's stress and recovery status.

Consumer Wearables Adapted for Dogs: Some pet owners have successfully used human wearable heart rate monitors (like Polar H10) adapted to fit their dog's chest, though this requires care for accuracy and comfort.

Observation of Behavior and Recovery: Since technology isn't always accessible, watching how quickly your dog recovers from stress—how calm they become after excitement or anxiety—can be an indirect indicator of healthy HRV and vagal tone.

By tracking HRV over time, either with technology or close observation, you can better understand your dog's internal stress levels and overall well-being.

Scientific Snippet:
According to research published in Frontiers in Veterinary Science, HRV monitoring can be used to assess welfare in dogs and identify stress. Vagal tone, assessed via HRV, reflects the dog's adaptability to changing environments.
https://www.frontiersin.org/articles/10.3389/fvets.2020.00634/full

Why This Matters

Understanding HRV as a marker of vagal tone can empower dog owners, trainers, and veterinarians to evaluate a dog's internal stress levels even before outward behavioral signs appear. This is especially important for dogs who are sensitive, fearful, rescue animals with traumatic backgrounds, or older dogs dealing with age-related stress.

Improving a dog's HRV—and therefore their vagal tone—can lead to reduced anxiety, improved digestion, better immune responses, and even enhanced learning and social behavior. That's how essential the vagus nerve is to your dog's emotional and physical life.

Chapter Sixteen

Breathing and Heart Rate

Breathing is not just a vital process that keeps your dog alive—it is a powerful tool for regulating emotional and physiological balance. In dogs, as in humans, the rhythm of the breath directly influences the vagus nerve and heart rate, both of which are integral to managing stress, fear, and relaxation.

When a dog is calm and breathing slowly and deeply, the vagus nerve is more active, promoting parasympathetic ("rest and digest") activity. This leads to a slower heart rate, relaxed muscles, steady digestion, and a calm demeanor. On the other hand, when a dog is frightened or anxious, breathing becomes shallow and rapid, and the vagus nerve becomes less active. This shifts the body into sympathetic mode, increasing heart rate and preparing the dog for fight-or-flight—an exhausting and harmful state when it persists too long.

The good news is that we can influence this system. While dogs can't be taught to consciously slow their breath like humans, we can guide their breath rhythm and vagus nerve tone by controlling their environment, routines, and physical touch. A relaxed environment, gentle massage, consistent routines, and time to decompress all encourage slower breathing and heart rate patterns, promoting vagal activity.

Breathing patterns are also closely tied to heart rate variability (HRV)—a vital measure of health. HRV is the variation in time between heartbeats. A higher HRV is associated with resilience and strong parasympathetic tone, while a low HRV indicates stress, fatigue, or illness. In dogs, increasing HRV is a goal that directly supports long-term health and behavior stability.

Research shows that vagal tone (the strength of the vagus nerve's influence) plays a critical role in heart rate regulation and emotional control. One study found that "vagal mechanisms are primary contributors to short-term HRV," meaning that stimulating the vagus nerve can lead to improvements in both mood and cardiovascular health.

Scientific Snippet: "Vagal mechanisms are the main contributors to the short-term variability of the heart rate."
Link to full study: https://pubmed.ncbi.nlm.nih.gov/10673367/

By using gentle techniques to calm your dog—like slow petting, massage along the neck and chest, allowing decompression walks, and creating safe spaces—you support healthier breathing, improved vagal tone, and ultimately a more emotionally balanced dog. The goal is not just to reduce anxiety, but to increase your dog's overall capacity for relaxation and resilience.

Conclusion

Embracing Your Dog's Natural Healing Power

As you reach the end of this book, I want to honor the incredible journey you and your dog have embarked on together. Understanding the vagus nerve and its profound influence on your dog's physical health, emotional balance, and behavior opens a beautiful door to natural healing and deep connection.

Your dog's nervous system is a remarkable gateway to wellness—an intricate network designed to keep them calm, resilient, and thriving even in the face of stress and challenges. By learning to support the vagus nerve through simple yet powerful techniques like touch, breath, sound, nutrition, and mindful routines, you are empowering your dog to access their own inner healing abilities.

This process is gentle and gradual. There is no rush or quick fix here—only consistent, compassionate care that honors your dog's unique needs and rhythms. The changes you foster may begin subtly: a calmer breath, a softer gaze, a quieter moment of peace—but over time, these small shifts build a foundation of lasting well-being.

Remember, the bond you share with your dog is central to this healing work. Your presence, patience, and love are as vital as any technique or tool. When you approach this with an open heart and steady commitment, you create a safe space where your dog feels truly seen, heard, and supported.

Challenges will come, as they do in any life, but with these practices in place, you both will be better equipped to navigate them with grace and resilience. Celebrate every step forward, no matter how small, knowing that you are helping your dog live a happier, more balanced life.

Thank you for your dedication to your dog's health and happiness. By embracing their natural healing power, you are not only enriching their life but deepening a lifelong partnership filled with trust, joy, and unconditional love.

Together, may you both continue to grow, heal, and thrive.

Bonus Section

Practical Tips to Support Your Dog's Vagus Nerve and Well-Being

Supporting your dog's vagus nerve function is a beautiful, ongoing journey that combines simple daily habits with mindful care. These practical tips can be incorporated into your dog's routine to enhance calm, reduce anxiety, and promote holistic health.

1. Consistent Daily Routine

Feed your dog at the same times every day to create predictability and reduce stress.

Schedule walks and play sessions consistently to balance physical activity and rest.

Maintain a regular bedtime routine to support healthy sleep cycles and vagal tone.

2. Gentle Touch and Massage

Practice slow, rhythmic strokes on your dog's ears, chest, and belly to stimulate vagal nerve endings.

Use soft pressure and pay attention to your dog's reactions—stop if they show discomfort.

Incorporate light acupressure on points near the neck and shoulders to ease tension.

3. Breath Synchronization

Practice slow, deep breathing while sitting calmly with your dog. Your steady breath rhythm can encourage their nervous system to relax in sync.

Try counting your breaths slowly (e.g., inhale for 4 seconds, exhale for 6) and observe your dog's calming response.

4. Create a Calming Sound Environment

Play soft classical music, nature sounds, or low-frequency tones during quiet times or stressful events like thunderstorms or fireworks.

Avoid loud, sudden noises that can trigger fight-or-flight responses.

5. Provide a Safe, Quiet Space

Designate a cozy corner or crate with soft bedding where your dog can retreat when overwhelmed.

Add familiar scents or a favorite toy to this area to make it feel secure.

6. Use Aromatherapy with Caution

Diffuse calming essential oils such as lavender or chamomile in a well-ventilated room (never apply oils directly to your dog).

Monitor for any signs of sensitivity or allergy and discontinue if adverse reactions occur.

7. Incorporate Moderate Exercise

Engage your dog in daily walks, swimming, or gentle play that promotes cardiovascular health without overexertion.

Tailor exercise intensity to your dog's age, breed, and fitness level to avoid stress from overdoing it.

8. Support Gut Health with Nutrition

Include probiotic-rich foods or supplements recommended by your vet to nurture a balanced microbiome.

Add omega-3 fatty acids (fish oil or plant-based alternatives) to your dog's diet to reduce inflammation and support nerve health.

Avoid processed treats with artificial additives that may disrupt gut and nervous system balance.

9. Mindful Interaction and Socialization

Spend quality time with calm, positive interactions—gentle petting, quiet companionship, and soft voices.

Facilitate positive social experiences with other dogs or trusted humans, respecting your dog's comfort level.

10. Use Technology Thoughtfully

Explore non-invasive vagus nerve stimulation devices under veterinary guidance if your dog has chronic anxiety or inflammation.

Track heart rate variability (HRV) with pet-friendly monitors to observe improvements in vagal tone over time.

11. Train with Patience and Positive Reinforcement

Use reward-based training methods that reduce stress and build confidence.

Avoid harsh corrections or unpredictable punishments that can activate fight-or-flight responses.

12. Monitor Stress Signals

Learn to recognize signs of stress such as yawning, lip licking, pacing, panting, or avoidance behaviors.

Intervene early by offering calming techniques or safe spaces to prevent chronic vagal dysfunction.

13. Use Vagal Activation Tools

Try slow, deliberate ear stroking or chest rubbing sessions daily.

Experiment with safe sound therapies or gentle vibration tools to stimulate vagal pathways.

14. Encourage Rest and Recovery

Ensure your dog has ample downtime after exercise or stimulating activities.

Create a low-stimulation environment for naps, promoting nervous system reset.

15. Hydration and Mineral Balance

Provide fresh water infused with appropriate electrolytes like potassium and magnesium (consult your vet).

Proper hydration supports nerve conductivity and overall vagal function.

16. Stay Patient and Consistent

Understand that improving vagal tone is a gradual process—results may take weeks or months to manifest.

Keep a journal of your dog's behavior, noting improvements or setbacks to share with your vet.

By integrating these tips into daily life, you empower your dog's natural ability to heal and maintain nervous system balance. Your love, attention, and consistency are the greatest gifts you can offer, fostering a calm, resilient, and joyful companion.

Thank You

From the bottom of my heart, thank you for choosing this book and taking the time to deepen your understanding of your dog's nervous system and natural healing power. Your commitment to learning about the vagus nerve and how to support it shows the deep love and care you have for your canine companion. It's people like you—dedicated, compassionate, and curious—who make the biggest difference in the lives of dogs everywhere.

This book is just the beginning of a journey toward greater connection, calm, and well-being for you and your dog. If you want to dive even deeper, I invite you to explore my Canine Vagus Nerve Activation Course available on my website. This course offers step-by-step guidance, practical demonstrations, and personalized tools to help you confidently apply vagal activation techniques at home.

Because you purchased this book, you're eligible for an exclusive 10% discount on the course as a special thank you. Simply visit the course page on my website:

https://payhip.com/INKEDEMOTIONS

Use the promo code13OKG2SNDZ at checkout to claim your savings.

Together, through knowledge and compassionate action, we can help dogs live happier, healthier, and more balanced lives. Thank you again for being part of this mission. I'm honored to support you and your dog every step of the way.

With gratitude and warm wishes,
Nikky Rich

Printed in Dunstable, United Kingdom